Jump Start

A Food Plan for Life

Eat Right
Move More
Journal Your Journey

It is that simple!

ISBN-13: 978-0692489291
ISBN-10: 0692489290

Dedicated to everyone who has tried and will try again and again and again...until they succeeds.

Table of Contents

Tips and Tricks

Season with salt while cooking but stop sprinkling your food at the table. You will get used to it.

Don't deprive yourself of anything. Nothing is off limits, but everything should be in moderation.

Take one day at a time.

It is about controlling your portions. Plain and simple.

Losing weight is not the end, it is the beginning.

Don't put anything off *until you lose weight*. You are spectacularly awesome just the way you are. Losing weight is not the goal, enjoying your fabulous life is the goal.

Love the food you eat.

Skipping sauces most of the time will generate amazing results – if you are a sauce person that is.

Vinegar rocks.

Track why you are eating and what you feel about food. It sounds simple, and a bit off perhaps, but it really works.

Be the person you want to be now, not the person you want to be when you are 10 pounds lighter.

You are as much about your perspective and attitude as you are about your weight. Remember this always.

Don't be hard on yourself. You are fabulously awesome always.

Spend five minutes an hour doing physical activity and track it.

Energy Out

Want to lose weight? The concept is relatively simple, the task, however, is not.

It all comes down to one thing, the energy expended each day must be greater than the calories, or energy, you take in. That really is all there is to it. For approximately every 3000 calories, give or take, you reduce – you will lose a pound.

This means, of course, there are no short cuts, no magic tricks, no hard and fast ways to lose weight – except one – eat less and move more.

This handbook is a combination food plan, recipe book and journal that will help you Jump Start your efforts, lose weight and feel good about your relationship with food. It is designed to help you be in control of what you eat – not the other way around.

A food plan is laid out for twenty days, complete with recipes. When the days are up, you may either repeat the entire program or substitute like dishes containing similar calorie counts. Go to my blog for more recipes and ideas.

The main thing is snacking. For the first 20 days the only snack allowable is an apple. Up to two per day. You may have them sliced, diced, whole, at one time, cut up or spaced out. It is up to you.

So what happens if you ditch the apple and eat a candy bar or a bag of chips, a big one, or a baker's dozen chewy gooey chocolate chip cookies? Absolutely nothing. You wash it down, whatever it is, with a big glass of water and you move on.

Remember: There is no better person to be than you, right here, right now!

Jump Start - Week 1-3

"Opportunities don't happen, you create them." --
Chris Grosser

Day 1

Breakfast:
- Hard boiled egg

Lunch:
- 1 Yoplait Light Yogurt
- Mix in ¼ cup granola
- Pour over 1/3 cup of fruit of your choice (I like berries)

Dinner:
- 1 whole chicken thigh – baked or grilled with paprika, salt and pepper – a pinch of garlic powder is also good
- 1 cup tossed pasta
    - boil pasta, let cool
    - add marinated artichoke hearts
    - celery
    - red peppers
    - salt and pepper to taste
- Salad with rice vinegar and pepper

Movement Journal - Moving Equals Energy Expended
How Much Did You Move Today?

Food notes and other thoughts for Day One

_____

_____

_____

_____

_____

_____

_____

Small Steps I've Made: _____

_____

_____

_____

_____

_____

_____

Blessings I Can Count: _____

_____

_____

_____

_____

_____

I attribute my success to this: I never gave or took any excuse.
–Florence Nightingale

Day 2

Breakfast:
- Hard boiled egg

Lunch:
- 1 Yoplait Light Yogurt
- Mix in ¼ cup granola
- Pour over 1/3 cup of fruit of your choice

Dinner:
- Large Chicken Salad
  - Cut 1 ½ of the leftover thighs and sprinkle with vinegar and ½ teaspoon of olive oil
  - Mix with lettuce and vegetables. Your salad fixings should equal two cups.
  - Add fruit ½ cup. Any fruit that is in season will work. I like strawberries or peaches. For crunch choose apples. Again, whatever is in season.

Movement Journal - Moving Equals Energy Expended
How Much Did You Move Today?

_____
_____
_____
_____
_____
_____
_____
_____
_____
_____

Food Thoughts and Other Notes for Day Two

_____

_____

_____

_____

_____

_____

_____

Small Steps I've Made: _____

_____

_____

_____

_____

_____

_____

Blessings I Can Count: _____

_____

_____

_____

_____

_____

Happiness depends upon ourselves.- Aristotle

Day 3

Breakfast:
- Hard boiled egg

Lunch:
- 1 Yoplait Light Yogurt
- Mix in ¼ cup granola
- Pour over 1/3 cup of fruit of your choice

Dinner:
- 6 ounces of grilled beef – steak, low fat hamburger, roast, tri tip any
- 1 ear of corn
- 1 baked potato with 1 teaspoon of butter and pepper
- ½ cup of fresh green beans sautéed with garlic and parsley

Movement Journal - Moving Equals Energy Expended
How Much Did You Move Today?

_____

_____

_____

_____

_____

_____

_____

_____

Food notes and other Thoughts for Day Three

_____

_____

_____

_____

_____

_____

_____

Small Steps I've Made: _____

_____

_____

_____

_____

_____

_____

_____

Blessings I Can Count: _____

_____

_____

_____

_____

_____

You miss 100% of the shots you don't take.
–Wayne Gretzky

Day 4

Breakfast:
- Hard boiled egg

Lunch:
- 1 Yoplait Light Yogurt
- Mix in ¼ cup granola
- Pour over 1/3 cup of fruit of your choice

Dinner:
- Chicken or beef burrito
    - Chop chicken or beef -- ¼ cup per person – I use leftover but you can use fresh
    - Heat up pan and cook meat until light brown
    - Add salsa and a pinch of brown sugar (or not)
    - Lightly salt
    - Add 1/8 to ¼ cup of water and reduce liquid
    - Grill tortilla – medium flour or corn
- Assemble burrito with cheese, red peppers, lettuce, onion, carrots – anything in moderation. The trick here is to have a medium burrito that wraps up, so fill it accordingly.
- Either a cup of refried beans or Spanish rice

Movement Journal - Moving Equals Energy Expended
How Much Did You Move Today?

Food notes and other Thoughts for Day Four

_____

_____

_____

_____

_____

_____

_____

Small Steps I've Made: _____

_____

_____

_____

_____

_____

_____

_____

Blessings I Can Count: _____

_____

_____

_____

_____

_____

The most difficult thing is the decision to act, the rest is merely tenacity.
–Amelia Earhart

Day 5

Breakfast:
- Hard boiled egg

Lunch:
- 1 Yoplait Light Yogurt
- Mix in ¼ cup granola
- Pour over 1/3 cup of fruit of your choice

Dinner
- Creamy Chicken or Shrimp Pasta
- 1 cup green vegetables
- 1 ½ cups of mixed salad with any vegetables – use vinegar dressing

Movement Journal – Moving Equals Energy Expended
How Much Did You Move Today?

Food notes and other Thoughts for Day Five

_____

_____

_____

_____

_____

_____

_____

Small Steps I've Made: _____

_____

_____

_____

_____

_____

_____

Blessings I Can Count: _____

_____

_____

_____

_____

_____

Every strike brings me closer to the next home run.
-Babe Ruth

Day 6

Breakfast:
- Hard boiled egg

Lunch:
- 1 Yoplait Light Yogurt
- Mix in ¼ cup granola
- Pour over 1/3 cup of fruit of your choice

Dinner:
- Grilled Hamburger – salt and pepper to taste
    - Lettuce, peppers, onion and tomatoes
    - Ketchup and / or mustard to taste
- ½ cup of pan fried potatoes
    - dice potatoes and red onion
    - heat pan, add one teaspoon of olive oil
    - add potatoes
    - salt and pepper to taste
- 1 cup green beans, sautéed with garlic and parsley

Movement Journal - Moving Equals Energy Expended
How Much Did You Move Today?

Food notes and other Thoughts for Day Six

_____

_____

_____

_____

_____

_____

_____

Small Steps I've Made: _____

_____

_____

_____

_____

_____

_____

_____

Blessings I Can Count: _____

_____

_____

_____

_____

_____

Definiteness of purpose is the starting point of all achievement.
–W. Clement Stone

Day 7

Breakfast:
- Hard boiled egg

Lunch:
- Peanut butter and jelly sandwich – 2 teaspoons of peanut butter only

Dinner:
- Wild card – eat what you want but no more than a cup of any starch

Movement Journal – Moving Equals Energy Expended
How Much Did You Move Today?

Food notes and other Thoughts for Day Seven

_____

_____

_____

_____

_____

_____

_____

Small Steps I've Made: _____

_____

_____

_____

_____

_____

_____

_____

Blessings I Can Count: _____

_____

_____

_____

_____

_____

We become what we think about.
–Earl Nightingale

Week One is Done!
Congratulations and celebrate your success.

How do you feel physically: _____

_____

_____

_____

How do you feel emotionally: _____

_____

_____

_____

List three successes of your first week? _____

_____

_____

_____

_____

_____

List something you would like to improve upon? _____

_____

_____

_____

_____

_____

Finish the following sentence: I am awesome because –

_____

_____

_____

_____

_____

_____

_____

Weight: _____

Time spent exercising: _____

Waist inches: _____

Hip inches: _____

If your clothes fit differently explain how: _____

_____

_____

The best thing that happened this week was: _____

_____

_____

_____

_____

Day 8

Breakfast:
- ½ to ¾ cup oatmeal and fruit

Lunch:
- 5 oz of white chicken meat
- Apple or melon

Dinner:
- Marmalade Chicken
- 1 cup green vegetable
- 2 cups salad

Movement Journal - Moving Equals Energy Expended
How Much Did You Move Today?

Food notes and other Thoughts for Day Eight

_____

_____

_____

_____

_____

_____

_____

Small Steps I've Made: _____

_____

_____

_____

_____

_____

_____

_____

Blessings I Can Count: _____

_____

_____

_____

_____

_____

Life is 10% what happens to me and 90% of how I react to it.
–Charles Swindoll

Day 9

Breakfast:
- Two scrambled eggs

Lunch:
- English muffin with 2 teaspoons almond butter
- Apple or melon

Dinner:
- Baked Chicken and Asparagus
- 2 cups salad – any vegetables, red bell peppers, onions, green bell peppers, lettuce, greens, snap peas, sprouts, tomatoes – anything raw and tasty

Movement Journal – Moving Equals Energy Expended
How Much Did You Move Today?

Food notes and other Thoughts for Day Nine

_____

_____

_____

_____

_____

_____

_____

Small Steps I've Made: _____

_____

_____

_____

_____

_____

_____

Blessings I Can Count: _____

_____

_____

_____

_____

_____

The most common way people give up their power is by thinking they don't have any. –Alice Walker

Day 10

Breakfast:
- Greek yogurt and a banana

Lunch:
- 1 cup of cut up Marmalade Chicken leftovers
- Apple or melon

Dinner:
- Sichuan Chicken
- 1 cup green vegetable
- 1 cup rice plain – white or brown
- 2 cups salad – any vegetables, red bell peppers, onions, green bell peppers, lettuce, greens, snap peas, sprouts, tomatoes – anything raw and tasty

Movement Journal – Moving Equals Energy Expended
How Much Did You Move Today?

Food notes and other Thoughts for Day Ten

_____

_____

_____

_____

_____

_____

_____

Small Steps I've Made: _____

_____

_____

_____

_____

_____

_____

Blessings I Can Count: _____

_____

_____

_____

_____

_____

The mind is everything. What you think you become.
–Buddha

Day 11

Breakfast:
- Hard boiled egg

Lunch:
- 1 Yoplait Light Yogurt
- Mix in ¼ cup granola
- Pour over 1/3 cup of fruit of your choice

Dinner:
- Chicken or beef burrito
    - Chop chicken or beef -- ¼ cup per person – I use leftover but you can use fresh
    - Heat up pan and cook meat until light brown
    - Add salsa and a pinch of brown sugar (or not)
    - Lightly salt
    - Add 1/8 to ¼ cup of water
    - Simmer to reduce liquid
    - Grill tortilla – medium flour or corn

Assemble burrito with cheese, red peppers, lettuce, onion, carrots – anything in moderation.

Movement Journal - Moving Equals Energy Expended
How Much Did You Move Today?

Food notes and other Thoughts for Day Eleven

_____

_____

_____

_____

_____

_____

_____

Small Steps I've Made: _____

_____

_____

_____

_____

_____

_____

_____

Blessings I Can Count: _____

_____

_____

_____

_____

_____

The best time to plant a tree was 20 years ago. The second best time is now. –Chinese Proverb

Day 12

Breakfast:
- ½ to ¾ cup oatmeal and fruit

Lunch:
- 4 oz of turkey
- 1 medium piece of fruit (apple, peach etc.)
- 1 English Muffin

Dinner:
- Crusted Chicken Salad With Pomegranate Balsamic Dressing
- 1 cup rice or 1 medium potato

Movement Journal - Moving Equals Energy Expended
How Much Did You Move Today?

Food Notes and Other Thoughts for Day Twelve

_____

_____

_____

_____

_____

_____

_____

Small Steps I've Made: _____

_____

_____

_____

_____

_____

_____

Blessings I Can Count: _____

_____

_____

_____

_____

_____

Whether you think you can or you think you can't, you're right.
–Henry Ford

Day 13

Breakfast:
- 2 eggs cooked anyway

Lunch:
- 5 oz of lean meat
- 1 medium piece of fruit (apple, peach etc.)
- ½ cup of quinoa – precooked.

Dinner:
- Chimichanga
- 2 cups salad

Movement Journal – Moving Equals Energy Expended
How Much Did You Move Today?

Food Notes and Other Thoughts for Day Thirteen

_____

_____

_____

_____

_____

_____

_____

Small Steps I've Made: _____

_____

_____

_____

_____

_____

_____

Blessings I Can Count: _____

_____

_____

_____

_____

_____

I am not a product of my circumstances. I am a product of my decisions.
–Stephen Covey

Day 14

Breakfast:
- Hard boiled egg

Lunch:
- 1 Yoplait Light Yogurt
- Mix in ¼ cup granola
- Pour over 1/3 cup of fruit of your choice

Dinner:
- Wild card – eat what you want but no more than a cup of any starch

Movement Journal – Moving Equals Energy Expended
How Much Did You Move Today?

Food Notes and Other Thoughts for Day Fourteen

_____

_____

_____

_____

_____

_____

_____

Small Steps I've Made: _____

_____

_____

_____

_____

_____

_____

_____

Blessings I Can Count: _____

_____

_____

_____

_____

_____

Life shrinks or expands in proportion to one's courage.
–Anais Nin

Week Two is Done!
Congratulations and celebrate your success.

How do you feel physically: _____

_____

_____

_____

_____

_____

How do you feel emotionally: _____

_____

_____

_____

List three successes of your second week? _____

_____

_____

_____

_____

_____

_____

List something you would like to improve on? _____

_____

_____

_____

_____

Finish the following sentence: I am awesome because –

_____

_____

_____

_____

_____

_____

_____

_____

Weight: _____

Time spent exercising: _____

Waist inches: _____

Hip inches: _____

If your clothes fit differently explain how: _____

_____

_____

_____

Use the space below to write about your thoughts when you just want to eat. In other words – write instead of eating something you may regret later. Explain what you want to eat and why. Dig deep and search for the real reasons you want to eat, because chances are you are not hungry. If you are hungry, have a piece of fruit and move on.

Notes, thoughts and things –

_____

_____

_____

_____

_____

_____

_____

_____

_____

_____

_____

_____

_____

_____

The best thing that happened this week was: _____

_____

_____

_____

_____

_____

_____

_____

Day 15

Breakfast:
- 2 boiled eggs and fruit

Lunch:
- 1 Yoplait Light Yogurt
- Mix in ¼ cup granola
- Pour over 1/3 cup of fruit of your choice

Dinner
- ½ cup of whole wheat pasta with marinara sauce
- 1 cup green vegetables
- 1 ½ cups of mixed salad with any vegetables – use vinegar dressing

Movement Journal – Moving Equals Energy Expended
How Much Did You Move Today?

Food Notes and Other Thoughts for Day Fifteen

_____

_____

_____

_____

_____

_____

_____

_____

Small Steps I've Made: _____

_____

_____

_____

_____

_____

_____

_____

Blessings I Can Count: _____

_____

_____

_____

_____

Go confidently in the direction of your dreams. Live the life you have imagined. –Henry David Thoreau

Day 16

Breakfast:
- 1 egg and English muffin

Lunch:
- 4 to 5 oz of turkey
- 1 medium piece of fruit (apple, peach etc.)
- 23 almonds

Dinner
- Chicken and Sprout Stir-fry
- ¾ cup rice – brown or white

List five things you like about the way you look:

1. _____

2. _____

3. _____

4. _____

5. _____

List five different ways you are going to move starting tomorrow:

1. _____

2. _____

3. _____

4. _____

5. _____

Food Notes and Other Thoughts for Day Sixteen

_____

_____

_____

_____

_____

_____

_____

Small Steps I've Made: _____

_____

_____

_____

_____

_____

_____

Blessings I Can Count: _____

_____

_____

_____

_____

_____

The only person you are destined to become is the person you decide to be. –Ralph Waldo Emerson

Day 17

Breakfast:
- 2 eggs or 1 cup of oatmeal
- English Muffin (omit muffin if you have oatmeal)

Lunch:
- 1 Yoplait Light Yogurt
- Mix in ¼ cup granola
- Pour over 1/3 cup of fruit of your choice

Dinner:
- Grilled Chicken Penne Pasta
- 1 cup green salad

Movement Journal – Moving Equals Energy Expended
How Much Did You Move Today?

Food Notes and Other Thoughts for Day Seventeen

_____

_____

_____

_____

_____

_____

_____

Small Steps I've Made: _____

_____

_____

_____

_____

_____

_____

_____

Blessings I Can Count: _____

_____

_____

_____

_____

_____

There is only one way to avoid criticism: do nothing, say nothing, and be nothing. –Aristotle

Day 18

Breakfast:
- Two scrambled eggs

Lunch:
- English muffin with 2 teaspoons almond butter
- Apple or melon

Dinner:
- Tomato Tart
- 1 cup green vegetables

Movement Journal - Moving Equals Energy Expended
How Much Did You Move Today?

Food Notes and Other Thoughts for Day Eighteen

_____

_____

_____

_____

_____

_____

_____

Small Steps I've Made: _____

_____

_____

_____

_____

_____

_____

Blessings I Can Count: _____

_____

_____

_____

_____

_____

Fall seven times and stand up eight.
–Japanese Proverb

Day 19

Breakfast:
- Greek yogurt and a banana

Lunch:
- 5 oz of turkey on an English Muffin
- Apple or melon

Dinner:
- Grilled Skirt Steak with Roasted Tomatillos
- 2 cups green salad

Movement Journal – Moving Equals Energy Expended
How Much Did You Move Today?

Food Notes and Other Thoughts for Day Nineteen

_____

_____

_____

_____

_____

_____

_____

Small Steps I've Made: _____

_____

_____

_____

_____

_____

_____

Blessings I Can Count: _____

_____

_____

_____

_____

_____

Too many of us are not living our dreams because we are living our fears.
–Les Brown

Day 20

Breakfast:
- 1 egg and 1 English muffin

Lunch:
- Almond butter and jelly sandwich – with two teaspoons each

Dinner:
- Wild card – eat what you want but no more than a cup of any starch

You did it!
You Successfully Completed the 20 Day Jump Start

Pat yourself on your back and continue to follow the pattern of healthy eating. The longer you do – the more ingrained the habit of healthy eating will be within you and the better you will feel.

If you still need the pattern of a daily menu planned out for you, the breakfasts, lunches and dinners in this book are designed to be mixed and matched! So have fun with them.

And don't forget your apple a day!

How does it feel to be successful? Remember success is that you put one foot in front of the other, took one day at a time and just did it. Concentrate on what worked.

_____

_____

_____

_____

_____

Week 3 and Phase One are Done!
Congratulations and Celebrate Your Success

How do you feel physically: _____

_____

_____

_____

_____

_____

How do you feel emotionally: _____

_____

_____

_____

List three successes of your first week? _____

_____

_____

_____

_____

_____

_____

List something you would like to improve on? _____

_____

_____

_____

_____

_____

Finish the following sentence: I am awesome because –

_____

_____

_____

_____

_____

_____

_____

_____

Weight: _____

Time spent exercising: _____

Waist inches: _____

Hip inches: _____

Explain the easiest part of this program for you: _____

_____

_____

_____

_____

Describe the most difficult part of the program for you:

_____

_____

_____

_____

Jump Start - Recipes

"It is never to late to be what you might have been."
-- George Eliot

Marmalade Chicken

Makes: 4 servings
Total Time: 20 minutes

INGREDIENTS

       1 cup chicken broth – homemade is best
       2 tablespoons red-wine vinegar
       2 tablespoons orange marmalade
       1 teaspoon lemon juice
       1 teaspoon cornstarch
       1 pound chicken tenders
       1/2 teaspoon salt
       1/4 teaspoon freshly ground pepper
       6 teaspoons olive oil
       2 large shallots, minced
       1 teaspoon freshly grated orange zest

PREPARATION

Mix broth, vinegar, marmalade, lemon and cornstarch in a medium bowl.

Sprinkle chicken with a touch of salt and pepper to taste. Heat 4 teaspoons oil in a large pan over medium-high heat. Add chicken – cook 2ish minutes per side. Remove chicken from pan and cover with foil to keep warm.

Add the remaining oil and shallots to pan and cook, stirring often. Cook for about 30 seconds. Mix the broth mixture and add it to the pan. Bring to a simmer, scraping any browned bits into the mixture.

Reduce heat to simmer; cook until the sauce is slightly reduced and thickened, a couple of minutes. Add chicken and return to a simmer. Cook until the chicken is heated throughout. Remove from the heat and stir in orange zest.

Grilled Salmon

Makes: Makes 4 servings
Total Time: 30 minutes

INGREDIENTS
> 2 cloves garlic, minced
> salt to taste
> 1 tablespoon olive oil
> 1 whole wild salmon fillet
> 1/3 cup plus 1/4 cup thinly sliced fresh basil, divided
> 2 medium tomatoes, thinly sliced
> ground pepper to taste

PREPARATION

Preheat grill to medium heat.

Mash garlic and 3/4 teaspoon salt with the a spoon until a paste forms.

Transfer to a small bowl and stir in oil.

Remove salmon pin bones If necessary. Cut a piece of foil large enough for the salmon fillet.

Spray the foil with fat free cooking spray. Place the salmon skin-side down on the foil and spread the garlic mixture on it. Sprinkle with crushed basil. Overlap tomato slices on top and sprinkle salt and pepper.

Put the salmon on the foil to the grill. Grill until salmon flakes easily. Usually 10 to 15 minutes.

Serve the salmon sprinkled with more basil.

For added zest – drizzle with lemon, lime or squeeze on a fresh mandarin or other citrus.

Sichuan Chicken

Makes: 4 servings, 1 cup each
Total Time: 25 minutes

INGREDIENTS

SICHUAN SAUCE

 3 tablespoons chicken broth
 1 tablespoon tomato paste
 2 teaspoons rice vinegar or balsamic vinegar
 1 teaspoon sugar
 1 teaspoon reduced-sodium soy sauce
 1/2 teaspoon sesame oil
 1/2 teaspoon brown sugar
 1/4 teaspoon cornstarch
 crushed red pepper to taste

CHICKEN

 1 pound skinless, boneless chicken breast, or thighs, trimmed and cut into 1-inch cubes
 1 teaspoon rice wine or sherry
 1 teaspoon reduced-sodium soy sauce
 1 1/2 teaspoons cornstarch
 1/2 teaspoon minced garlic
 1 tablespoon olive oil
 2 1/2-inch-thick slices ginger, minced
 2 cups sugar snap peas: fresh or frozen
 1/4 cup dry-roasted or honey roasted peanuts
 1 scallion, minced

PREPARATION

Sichuan sauce: Mix broth, tomato paste, vinegar, sugar, soy sauce, sesame oil, cornstarch, brown sugar and crushed red pepper to taste in a bowl.

Chicken: Combine chicken, rice wine (or sherry), soy sauce, cornstarch and garlic in another bowl. Mix well.

Heat a wok or large skillet over high heat.

Warm oil in pan, add ginger and stir-fry for 10 seconds.

Add the chicken, spreading it out in the pan to cook well.

Cook until the chicken begins to brown, 1ish minute.

Using a spatula or flat wooden spoon, stir-fry for 30 seconds.

Spread the chicken out again and cook for 30 seconds.

Continue stir-frying until the chicken is lightly browned on all sides, 1 to 2 minutes.

Add snap peas and cook for another minute or two.

Stir the Sichuan sauce, add to pan and stir-fry until chicken is cooked through and the sauce is slightly thickened – 30 seconds to 1 minute and 30 seconds.

Put on plate and sprinkle with scallions and nuts.

My Cooking Notes

Creamy Chicken (or Shrimp) Pasta

Makes: 4 servings, about 2 cups each
Total Time: 30 minutes

INGREDIENTS
>   6 oz whole-wheat angel hair
>   12 oz white chicken meat (or shrimp)
>   1 bunch asparagus, thinly sliced
>   1 large red bell pepper, thinly sliced
>   1 cup peas
>   3 cloves garlic, chopped
>   1 1/4 teaspoons salt
>   1 1/2 cups nonfat or low-fat plain yogurt
>   1/4 cup chopped flat-leaf parsley
>   3 tablespoons lemon juice
>   1 tablespoon extra-virgin olive oil
>   1/2 teaspoon freshly ground pepper
>   1/4 cup toasted pine nuts

PREPARATION

Cook pasta, drain and put back in pot.

Add shrimp or chicken, asparagus, bell pepper and peas and cook until the pasta is tender and the shrimp or chicken are cooked. Approximately, 2 to 4 minutes more.

Mash garlic and salt in a large bowl until a paste forms.

Mix in yogurt, parsley, lemon juice, oil and pepper.

Add the pasta mixture and toss until sauce covers.

Serve sprinkled with pine nuts.

For zestier recipe use Greek yogurt instead of regular.

Breadcrumb Crusted Chicken Salad With Pomegranate Balsamic Dressing

Makes: 4 servings, about 2 cups each
Total Time: 30 minutes

INGREDIENTS
>   4 boneless skinless chicken breast halves
>   salt and pepper to taste
>   3 eggs, beaten
>   1 1/2 tablespoons water
>   4 cups breadcrumbs
>   5 tablespoons olive oil
>   4 cups mixed greens, washed and dried

Caramelized Fruit
>   2 firm plums
>   2 firm peaches
>   2 firm nectarines
>   1 teaspoon olive oil

If fresh fruit is unavailable, you may use frozen

Pomegranate Balsamic Dressing
>   3/4 cup pomegranate juice
>   1/4 cup balsamic vinegar
>   2 tablespoons honey
>   3 tablespoons orange or pineapple juice
>   1/4 cup olive oil

PREPARATION

Place chicken between 2 sheets of plastic wrap and pound to approximately 1/2 inch thickness.

Salt and pepper to taste. In a flat bowl, beat eggs and stir in water. Put breadcrumbs in another dish.

Dip each chicken breast in egg mixture, let excess drip off and then place in breadcrumbs. Coat both sides of chicken with breadcrumbs.

Place olive oil in pan over medium high heat.

Add chicken and cook 8 to 10 minutes, turning once.

Remove chicken from pan and cut into strips.

On each of the serving plates, place greens and top with chicken. Add Caramelized Fruit and drizzle with dressing

Caramelized Fruit:
Cut fruit into halves - remove pits. Cut pitted fruit into wedges.

Heat pan over medium heat.

Add fruit and cook 3 minutes on each side, until fruit starts to turn brown and caramelize.

Remove from heat and set aside.

Pomegranate Balsamic Dressing:
Cook 3/4 cup pomegranate juice and 1/4 cup balsamic vinegar in a medium pan.

Cook about 15 to 25 minutes, stirring often. Cook until syrupy.

Stir in honey and 3 tablespoons orange or pineapple juice and simmer about 7 minutes.

Remove from heat and stir in 1/2 cup olive oil.

Oven Fried Chicken Chimichangas

Makes: 4 servings
Total Time: 20 minutes

INGREDIENTS

- 2/3 cup salsa
- 1 teaspoon ground cumin
- 1/2 teaspoon dried oregano leaves, crushed
- 1 1/2 cups cooked chicken, chopped
- 1 cup shredded cheddar cheese
- 2 green onions, chopped with some tops (about 1/4 cup)
- 6 (8 inch) flour tortillas
- at free cooking spray

  shredded cheddar cheese
- chopped green onion
- picante or more salsa sauce

PREPARATION

Mix chicken, salsa, cumin, oregano, cheese and onions.

Place about 1/4 ish cup of the chicken mixture in each of the tortillas.

Fold tortilla.

Roll up from bottom and place open-side down on a baking sheet.

Spray with fat free cooking spray.

Bake at 400°F for 25 minutes or until golden.

Add additional cheese and green onion and serve salsa on the side.

Oregano and Lemon Kebabs

Makes: 4 servings
Total Time: 20 minutes

INGREDIENTS
  1 b lean pork loin, cut into cubes or chicken

Marinade

  1/2 cup lemon juice
  1 tablespoon oil
  2 teaspoons oregano
  1 teaspoon rosemary
  1 garlic clove, crushed
  fresh ground black pepper
  1 medium red pepper, cut into large chunks
  1 medium zucchini, cut into thick slices
  8 cherry tomatoes, green grape preferred
  1 medium onion, cut into large chunks
  8 medium white mushrooms

PREPARATION

Marinade: Combine all ingredients in a reusable plastic bag.

Trim meat and cut into 1 inch cubes.

Place meat in bag and marinate in the refrigerator fridge for 30 minutes to overnight.

Soak wooden skewers in water and wash and cut vegetables for kebabs.

Make kebabs alternating between the meat and vegetables.

Place on grill and cook for approximately 10 minutes.

Chicken and Sprouts Stir Fry

Makes: 4 servings
Total Time: 32 minutes

INGREDIENTS

    4 boneless skinless chicken breasts
    2 cups bean sprouts
    2 1/2 tablespoons vegetable oil
    1 1/2 teaspoon ginger, minced
    2 garlic cloves, minced
    3/4 cup scallion, chopped
    3/4 cup carrot, chopped
    3/4 cup red bell peppers, chopped
    4 tablespoons reduced sodium soy sauce
    3 tablespoons honey

PREPARATION

In a large pan, heat 1 1/2 tablespoons oil. Add sprouts and cook, stir until lightly browned and tender, 1 to 2 minutes.

Transfer sprouts and cover to keep warm.

Add remaining oil to the same pan and heat for 1 minute; add chicken, garlic, carrots, red peppers and ginger and stir-fry for 3 minutes.

Add scallions and continue cooking until chicken is tender and browned on all sides, 2 to 3 minutes longer.

Add soy sauce (to taste) and honey; cook, stirring constantly for approximately 1 minute longer.

Put warm chicken mixture on plates and top with sprouts.

Grilled Chicken Bow-tie Pasta

Makes: 4 servings
Total Time: 32 minutes

INGREDIENTS

    2 chicken breasts, grilled and sliced
    1/2 medium yellow onion, finely chopped
    4 garlic cloves, minced
    1 (14 1/2 ounce) can tomatoes, diced
    1 (14 1/2 ounce) can tomato sauce
    1 (6 ounce) can tomato juice
    2 medium tomatoes
    2 tablespoons fresh basil chopped
    1 tablespoon olive oil
    1 oregano
    1 tablespoon parsley, chopped fresh
    salt and pepper to taste
    2 cups bow-tie paste

PREPARATION

Sauté onions in olive oil.

Add garlic and cook for about 1 more minute.

Add tomato, tomato sauce, tomato juice, black pepper, salt, basil, and parsley.

Bring sauce to a boil and then reduce to simmer and add grilled chicken.

Cut whole tomatoes and swirl into pan chicken mixture.

Cook penne pasta in boiling, salted water. Strain pasta and add to sauce.

Sprinkle with oregano.

Tomato Tart

Makes: 4 servings
Total Time: 32 minutes

INGREDIENTS
>1/2 (14.1-ounce) package refrigerated pie dough
>Cooking spray
>1 cup ounces shredded cheese
>1/2 cup pitted olives, chopped
>1/3 cup sliced shallots
>3 tomatoes, cut into 1/2-inch-thick slices
>3 tablespoons flour
>1 tablespoon cornmeal
>1 tablespoon thyme
>1 1/4 cups 2% reduced-fat milk
>1 1/2 tablespoons grated Parmesan
>3 large eggs
>2 tablespoons fresh basil leaves
>1 cup cherry tomatoes, quartered

PREPARATION
Preheat oven to 350°.

Coat pay pan with non-fat cooking spray. Roll dough and press into a 9-inch deep-dish pan.

Sprinkle with cheese, olives, and shallots.

Arrange half of tomato slices over above.

Combine flour, cornmeal, and thyme; sprinkle over tomatoes. Top with remaining tomato slices.

Mix milk, Parmesan, and eggs; pour into pan. Bake for 40 minutes or until set; let stand 10 minutes.

Top with basil and rest of tomatoes.

Grilled Skirt Steak with Roasted Tomatillo Sauce

Makes: 4 servings
Total Time: 32 minutes

INGREDIENTS
>   1 cup boiling water
>   1 dried chile, stemmed
>   3 tablespoons chopped fresh oregano, divided
>   2 tablespoons fresh lime juice, divided
>   1 tablespoon olive oil
>   1 1/2 teaspoons ground cumin, divided
>   8 garlic cloves, divided
>   1 (1-pound) skirt steak, trimmed
>   1/2 cup sliced green or yellow onion
>   8 ounces tomatillos, husks removed
>   Salt and pepper to taste
>   Pinch of sugar
>   2 tablespoons chopped fresh cilantro

PREPARATION

Preheat oven to 450°.

Steep chile in 1 cup boiling water and let stand 10 minutes or until hydrated. Drain and finely chop .

Combine chile, oregano, juice, oil, and cumin in a plastic bag. Mince 4 garlic cloves and add to bag. Add steak to bag. Shake to fully coat.

Refrigerate for and hour to an hour and 1/2.

Mince remaining garlic cloves. Place minced garlic, onions and tomatillos i on a baking sheet coated with non-gat cooking spray.

Bake at 450° for 20 minutes.

Combine tomatillo mixture, remaining 2 tablespoons oregano, remaining 1 tablespoon juice, remaining 1/2 teaspoon cumin, salt, pepper and sugar in a blender; mix until smooth, scraping sides.

Preheat grill to high.

Remove steak from bag; sprinkle both sides of meat evenly with remaining salt and pepper. Place steak on grill rack coated with cooking spray. Grill until done.

My Cooking Notes

Meatloaf with Mozzarella and Mushrooms

Makes: 4 servings
Total Time: 1.5 hours

INGREDIENTS

2 slices bread
1 1/2 pounds lean ground beef
1 cup shredded part-skim mozzarella
1/3 cup finely chopped pepperoni or salami
1 teaspoon dried oregano
1 teaspoon garlic powder
3/4 teaspoon salt
2 large eggs, lightly beaten
2 tablespoons ketchup

PREPARATION

Preheat over to 350 degrees.

Toast bread, blend to crumbs. Combine crumbs, beef, mozzarella, pepperoni, oregano, garlic, salt and eggs in a large bowl and mix gently with your hands to combine.

Form mixture into a 9-inch-by-6-inch loaf.

Brush meatloaf with ketchup, cover, and cook 1 hour.

Pair With:
- 2 cups salad with any vegetables
- 1 medium potato
- green vegetables

Chicken Cutlets with Mushrooms, Peppers and Mozzarella

Makes: 8 servings
Total time: 35 Minutes

INGREDIENTS

1/4 cup olive oil
1/4 cup flour
2 large eggs, lightly beaten
1 cup seasoned bread crumbs
8 boneless, skinless chicken breast halves
Salt and pepper
1 cup sliced mushrooms
1/4 cup white wine
1 7.5-oz. jar roasted red peppers, drained, cut into strips
8 ounces sliced mozzarella

PREPARATION

Preheat oven to 400°F.

Spray 9-by-13-inch with non-fat cooking spray. Place flour, eggs and bread crumbs in separate shallow bowls.

Season chicken with salt and pepper and dip in flour. Dip chicken in eggs and then dip in breadcrumbs. Place breaded chicken on a dish or tray.

Heat 1-tablespoon oil in a large pan over medium heat. Brown chicken, not all at once, flipping once, 2 to 3 minutes per side, adding more oil to pan between groups. Transfer browned chicken to baking dish.

In same pan, cook mushrooms, stirring, until golden brown, about 5 minutes.

Drizzle wine over meat, then top with mushrooms, peppers and cheese.

Bake chicken for 15 to 20 minutes.

Baked Chicken and Asparagus

Makes: 2 servings
Total Time: 50 minutes

INGREDIENTS
    1 whole boneless, skinless chicken breast
    8 oz jar of sun-dried tomatoes in olive oil
    Fresh Blanched asparagus
    Garlic-minced
    salt and pepper

PREPARATION

Put cleaned skinless chicken breast into a baking dish.

Blanch Asparagus and add to baking dish. Add sun-dried tomatoes, garlic and vegetables to the top of chicken.

Cover with foil.

Bake at 350 degrees for 50 minutes or until done.

Salt and pepper to taste.

Cooking Notes:

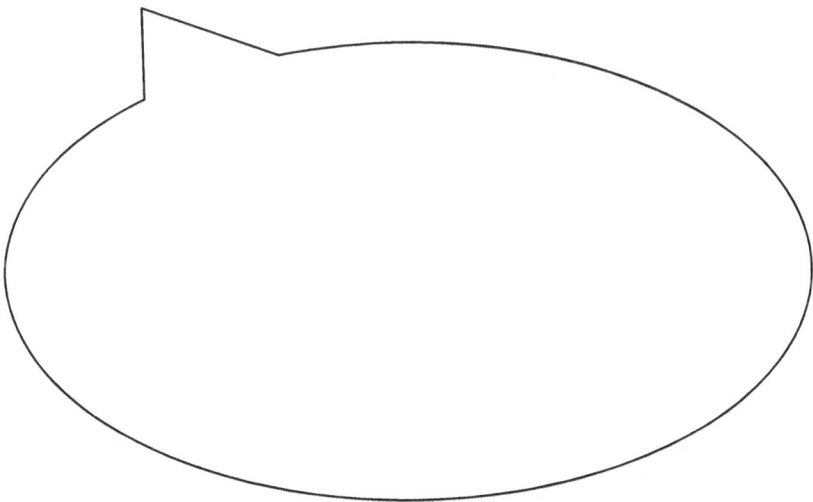

Whole Wheat Pasta with Sesame Peanut Sauce

Makes: 4 servings
Total Time: 20 minutes

INGREDIENTS

> 2 medium green onions, sliced thinly
> 1/4 cup chicken or vegetable broth
> 2 teaspoon peanut butter
> 1 Tablespoon plus 1 teaspoon cider vinegar
> 1 teaspoon sesame oil
> 1/4 to 1/2 teaspoon cayenne
> 4 cups cooked whole wheat spaghetti

PREPERATION

Combine all ingredients, MINUS pasta.

Stir the hot spaghetti into the sauce. Serve right away.

Serve With:

Snow Pea Salad

Makes: 4 servings
Total Time: 10 minutes

INGREDIENTS

> 1 cup fresh snow peas
> 1 cup bean sprouts
> 4 cups any type of lettuce
> 2 mandarin oranges, peeled and split
> onion
> rice vinegar – I like basil rice vinegar
> drizzle of olive oil

Mix ingredients and drizzle with dressing.

Grilled Cheese and Pizza Sandwich

Makes: 1 serving (double for 2)
Total Time: 10 minutes

INGREDIENTS
2 slices mixed grain bread
2 tablespoons marinara sauce
1/4 cup mozzarella cheese (low moisture, part skim)
1 teaspoon shredded Parmesan
Salt and pepper to taste

PREPARATION

Smear about 1 tablespoon of marinara sauce on each piece of bread. Sprinkle mozzarella cheese evenly over sauce. Sprinkle with Parmesan. Top with second piece of bread, sauce side down.

Place in heated pan and cook until cheese inside is melted and outside is golden brown.

Serve With:
Sweet Potato Fries

Makes: 4 servings
Total Time: 40 minutes

1 tbsp olive oil
2 5" long sweet potatoes

PREPARATION

Peel and cut sweet potatoes. Place in 9x13" pan and drizzle with olive oil.

Toss to coat evenly. Bake 35 minutes at 400 °F turning once.

Warm Sausage and Potato Salad

Makes: 4 servings
Total Time: 30 minutes

INGREDIENTS

> 1 pound small potatoes, cut in half
> 1 5-ounce bag arugula (about 4 cups, gently packed)
> 12 ounces sausage – cut in slices
> 1/3 cup cider vinegar
> 1 tablespoon maple syrup
> 1 tablespoon extra-virgin olive oil
> Freshly ground pepper, to taste

PREPARATION

Boil potatoes until cooked but not mushy.

Transfer to a large bowl and add arugula; cover with foil to keep warm.

Cook sausage in a medium pan over medium heat, until browned and heated throughout, about 5 minutes. Add to the potato-arugula mixture.

Remove the pan from the heat and mix in vinegar and maple syrup, scraping up any browned bits. Sprinkle with oil.

Pour dressing over the salad and toss until the arugula is wilted.

Season with pepper.

Hawaiian Ginger-Chicken Stew

Makes: 2 servings, about 1 cup each
Total Time: 35 minutes

INGREDIENTS
    1 1/2 teaspoons sesame oil
    1/2 pound chicken tenders
    1 1-inch piece fresh ginger, peeled and cut into matchsticks or minced
    2 cloves garlic, thinly sliced
    1/4 cup dry sherry
    1 cup chicken broth
    3/4 cup water
    1 tablespoon reduced-sodium soy sauce
    1/2 teaspoon Asian red chile sauce
    1/2 bunch mustard greens, or chard, stemmed and chopped (3-3 1/2 cups),

PREPARATION

Heat oil in a large saucepan over medium-high heat. Add chicken and cook, until just cooked through, about 6 minutes. Transfer to a plate.

Add ginger and garlic to the pot and cook about 10 seconds. Add sherry and cook until mostly reduced, scraping up any browned bits.

Add broth and water, increase heat to high and bring to a boil. Boil for 5 minutes. Add soy sauce, chile sauce and mustard greens (or chard) and cook until the greens are tender.

Return the chicken and any juices to the pot and cook until heated through, 1 to 2 minutes.

Salisbury Steak

Makes: 2 servings, about 1 cup each
Total Time: 35 minutes

INGREDIENTS

1 1/2 pounds of ground round
1/3 cup dry breadcrumbs
2 large egg whites
3/4 cup water
4 tablespoons tomato paste
2 tablespoons dry sherry
1 1/2 teaspoons Worcestershire sauce
1/4 teaspoon freshly ground black pepper
1 (10 1/2-ounce) can condensed French onion soup low-fat

PREPARATION

Combine meat and breadcrumbs. Divide into 6 equal portions, shaping each into a 1/2-inch-thick patty.

Heat a large nonstick skillet coated with cooking spray over medium-high heat.

Add patties; cook 5 to 6 minutes or until brown.

Remove patties from pan; keep warm. Stir in water and remaining ingredients. Bring to a boil; add patties.

Cover, reduce heat, and simmer 10 minutes.

Uncover and cook until wine mixture liquid in pay is reduced.

Balsamic Pork Chops

Makes: 4 servings
Total Time: 20 minutes

INGREDIENTS
    4 4 ounces. boneless pork chops
    2 teaspoon lemon pepper
    ½ cup balsamic vinegar
    ½ cup vegetable broth
    Salt and pepper to taste

PREPARATION

Salt and pepper meat

Spray a nonstick skillet with non-fat cooking spray and warm over medium high heat.

Add meat and cook until lightly browned, usually 4 to 5 minutes.

Remove from skillet and keep warm.

Wipe pan clean and then add vinegar and broth.

Cook about seven minutes or until sauce has reduced and thickened. Spoon over chops and serve immediately.

Serve With:
- White rice
- Green vegetables

Turkey Panini

Makes: 4 servings
Total Time: 20 minutes

INGREDIENTS

     3 tablespoons Greek yogurt
     2 tablespoons plain yogurt
     2 tablespoon shredded cheese
     2 tablespoon chopped basil
     1 teaspoon lemon juice
     8 slices light whole wheat bread
     8 oz. thinly sliced deli turkey
     8 slices tomato

PREPARATION

Mix Greek yogurt, yogurt, cheese, basil, lemon juice and pepper.

Spread 2 teaspoons of the mixture on each slice of bread and then fill the sandwiches with turkey and tomato.

Heat 1 teaspoon of oil in a large pan and put in 2 sandwiches.

Use a Panini press to weight down the sandwiches.

Cook until golden. Flip and do the same.

Cooking Notes:

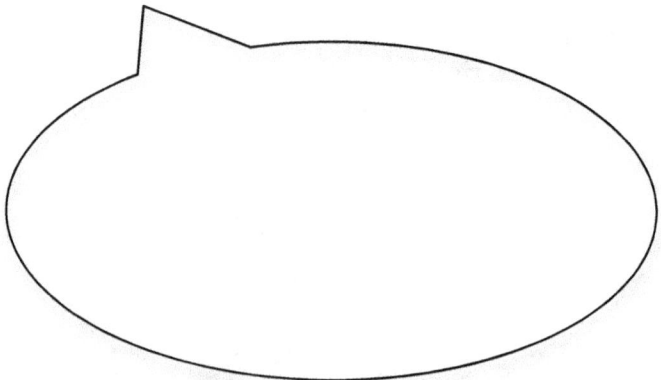

Pork and Soba Noodles

Makes: Serves 4
Total Time: 20 minutes

INGREDIENTS
>6 ounces soba noodles
>1 1 1/4-pound pork tenderloin, thinly sliced
>salt and black pepper
>1 tablespoon vegetable oil
>1/2 cucumber, sliced
>2 scallions, chopped
>1/2 cup of fresh snow peas
>1 red chili pepper, sliced
>2 tablespoons rice vinegar
>2 teaspoons sesame oil

PREPARATION

Cook the soba noodles.

Salt and pepper meat to taste

Heat oil in a large skillet over medium-high heat.

Brown the pork in batches, 2 to 3 minutes per side. Transfer to a large bowl.

Toss the pork with the noodles, cucumber, scallions, snow peas chili pepper, vinegar, sesame oil, and ½ teaspoon salt.

Cooking Notes:

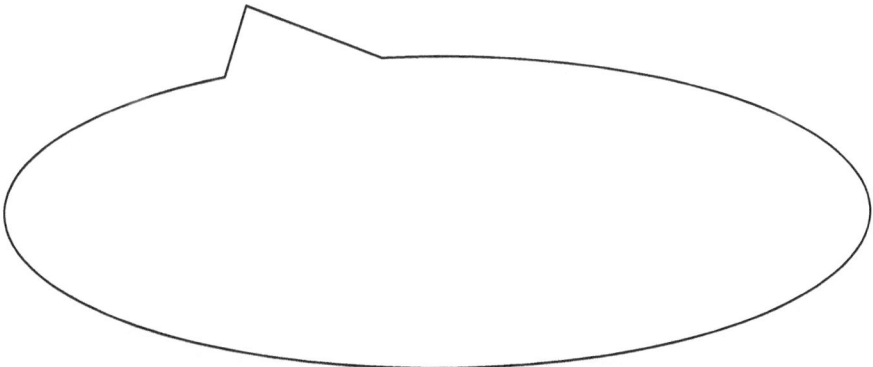

Mango Steak Salad

Makes: 4 servings
Total Time: 30 minutes

INGREDIENTS

      3/4 pound sirloin steak (1 inch thick)
      salt and black pepper
      1 teaspoon grated lime zest
      4 tablespoons fresh lime juice
      2 tablespoon honey
      2 teaspoons of apple cider vinegar
      2 teaspoons low-sodium soy sauce
      3 tablespoons olive oil
      1 large head romaine lettuce, cut into strips
      1 mango, cut into thin strips
      1 red bell pepper, thinly sliced
      1/2 cup fresh basil leaves, sliced
      2 scallions, thinly sliced
      1 teaspoon toasted sesame seeds

PREPARATION

Heat a large skillet over high heat.

Season the steak with salt and pepper. Cook 4 to 5 minutes per side for medium-rare. Let rest at least 5 minutes before slicing.

Mix together lime zest and juice, honey, apple cider vinegar, soy sauce, oil, and ¼ teaspoon salt. Add the lettuce, mango, bell pepper, basil, and scallions and toss to combine.

Gently fold in steak and sprinkle with the sesame seeds.

Sweet Basil, Tomato, Peach and Chicken Salad

Makes: 6 servings
Total Time: 20 minutes

INGREDIENTS
> 3 cups left over chicken, cut up or pulled into bit size pieces
> 4 Tablespoons balsamic vinegar
> 2 Tablespoons white balsamic or rice vinegar
> 2 teaspoons olive oil
> Black pepper
> 3 medium peaches, pitted and sliced
> 4 tomatoes, sliced horizontally or cut into wedges
> ¾ cup fresh basil, torn or coarsely chopped.

PREPARATION

Soak chicken bits in white balsamic or rice vinegar.

Mix oil, 4 Tablespoon balsamic vinegar and black pepper in a small bowl.

Place tomatoes and peaches on a platter or individual plates.

Pour on mixed oil, vinegar and black pepper. Sprinkle on chicken and sweet basil.

Quick and Creamy Pesto Pasta

Makes: 4 servings
Total Time: 30 minutes

INGREDIENTS
> 3 cups sweet basil crushed
> 2 Tablespoons olive oil
> ¼ cup non or low fat Greek yogurt
> salt, pepper and roasted pine nuts to taste
> 6 oz boiled pasta – shells

Cook pasta, mix in crushed basil, olive oil and Greek yogurt. Salt, pepper and roasted pine nuts to your liking.

Grilled Chicken and Green Beans

Makes: 4 servings
Total Time: 40 minutes

INGREDIENTS
 1 cup of low or non-fat Greet yogurt
 6 cloves of garlic
 10 pieces of bone in chicken pieces (I like thighs)
 salt, pepper and paprika to taste

PREPARATION

Combine Greek yogurt, garlic, salt, pepper and paprika in a small mixing bowl.

Put chicken in one or two large reusable close top plastic bags. Pour in yogurt mixture and swish. Put in refrigerate to marinate one hour to overnight.

Heat grill to medium or high medium. Remove chicken from marinate and grill until done.

Maple Green Beans

Makes: 4 servings
Total Time: 15 minutes

INGREDIENTS
 ½ cup pecans or almonds
 2 to 2 ½ pounds of green beans
 4 Tablespoons of olive oil
 2 Tablespoon balsamic vinegar
 1 Tablespoon maple syrup

PREPARATION

Roast nuts at 400 degrees for 5 to 7 minutes. Bring stock pot of water to boil and add salt. Toss in beans and cook until tender, but not mushy. About four minutes. Drain and run under cool water. Mix all ingredients in large bowl and serve.

Rice Over Easy

Makes: 4 servings
Total Time: 30 minutes

INGREDIENTS
>   2 Tablespoons olive oil
>   4 eggs, large or extra large
>   2 cloves of garlic, chopped
>   1 Tablespoon fresh ginger, chopped
>   6 oz fresh snow peas
>   6 cups of greens, cut (bok choy, chard or other)
>   3 ½ cups cooked brown rice
>   1 Tablespoon lemon juice
>   2 carrots, sliced
>   2 scallions, sliced

PREPARATION

Heat oil over medium heat in a large pan. Add eggs and season with salt and pepper. Cook (fry) until whites have crispy edges – 4 to 5 minutes. Remove from pan.

In same pan, put garlic, ginger, peas and greens, stir-fry for about 2 to 3 minutes. Add ¼ cup of water and reduce liquid.

Add rice and lemon juice. Mix.

Add carrots and scallions. Stir and cook until rice is warm. Season with salt and pepper to taste and serve hot.

Cooking Notes:

Milanish Summer Vegetable Pasta

Makes: 8 servings
Total Time: 40 minutes

INGREDIENTS

    3 Tablespoons olive oil
    1 medium summer squash, cut into chunks
    1 medium zucchini, cut into chunks
    1 medium eggplant, peeled and cut into chunks
    1 medium red onion, chopped
    1 to 2 cups chard, chopped
    2 cups fresh mushrooms, sliced
    2 cloves of garlic, finely minced
    2 pinches crushed red pepper
    1 can crushed tomatoes 28 oz
    ¼ cup sweet basil, chopped
    1 head parsley chopped
    2 Tablespoons fresh oregano, chopped
    1 package of whole wheat pasta – bows are fun

PREPARATION

Heat 1 T oil in a medium stockpot. Add zucchini, squash and cook until tender but not mushy. Remove.

In same pot, add 1 T oil and cook egg plant, mushrooms and onions. Add parsley, garlic and pepper flakes.

Add tomatoes, salt and pepper.

Stir in oregano and half of sweet basil. Reduce heat to low and cook for 15 minutes.

Cook pasta while vegetables are stewing.

Drain pasta and add to mixture. Top with shredded Parmesan cheese and the rest of the olive oil. Sprinkle remaining sweet basil.

Serve hot.

Chicken and Peach (or Mango) Fry

Makes: 4 servings
Total Time: 25 minutes

INGREDIENTS
>   3 large boneless chicken breasts
>   2 Tablespoons olive oil
>   salt and pepper
>   red pepper flakes
>   6 oz angel hair pasta, uncooked
>   2 to 3 cups snap peas
>   1 red bell pepper
>   1 yellow bell pepper
>   1/3 cup peach preserves
>   ¼ cup reduced sodium soy sauce
>   1 ½ Tablespoons brown sugar
>   1 clove of garlic
>   1 cup chopped peaches (or mangos)
>   ¼ cup cashews or walnuts, chopped

PREPARATION

Boil pasta according to directions on package

Cut chicken and salt, pepper and pepper flakes to taste.

Heat pan over medium heat. Cook chicken 3 to 4 minutes. Remove from pan.

Stir-fry snap peas, red peppers and yellow peppers in remaining olive oil until just tender, but still crunchy.

Stir in preserves, soy sauce and sugar.

Return chicken to pan and add peaches (or mangos).

Stir in pasta, top with nuts and serve piping hot.

Meatballs and Polenta

Makes: 4 servings
Total Time: 25 minutes

INGREDIENTS
     1 ½ cups of polenta
     1 pound of lean hamburger
     1 egg
     ¼ cup shredded Parmesan cheese
     3 Tablespoons sweet basil, chopped
     2 Tablespoons oregano, chopped
     salt and pepper to taste
     2 cups basic marinara sauce

PREPARATION

Pre-heat oven to 350 degrees.

Mix hamburger, egg, cheese, sweet basil, oregano, salt and pepper. Form into balls.

Spray a jelly roll pan or cooking sheet with non-fat cooking spray. Put meatballs on pan and bake for 20 minutes or until golden brown.

While the meatballs are cooking, cook polenta and warm marinara sauce.

Divide polenta onto plates, add meatballs and cover with marinara sauce.

Modifications:

- Add ½ Parmesan cheese to meatballs and sprinkle the rest of the cheese over plated meatballs.
- Slice polenta, add sauce and meatballs and put in over for 10 minutes
- Exchange Parmesan cheese for mozzarella

My Weight Loss Journal

Current Weight: _____ Date: _____

Goal Weight: _____ Date: _____

My Fitness Motto: _____

_____

_____

_____

Do Something Today That Your
Future Self Will Thank You For

Small goals for the duration of phase one of "Jump Start":

_____

_____

_____

_____

_____

_____

_____

_____

_____

_____

_____

_____

_____

_____

YOU DID IT DAY!!!

Now take a few minutes and plan out your next twenty days!

_____

_____

_____

_____

_____

_____

_____

_____

_____

_____

_____

_____

_____

_____

_____

_____

_____

_____

_____

_____

_____

_____

_____

Food for Thought

What Does 100 Calories Look Like
- 1 small potato – about 2 inches in diameter
- 1 ounce of cheddar cheese – low fat
- 9 spears of broccoli
- 12 Brussels Sprouts: plain
- 14 large shrimp – broiled
- 7 cashews
- 16 stalks of celery
- About 23 cloves of garlic
- 30 asparagus spears
- 33 grapes
- 60 raw green beans
- 82 canned beans, kidney
- About 100 raspberries
- 1 fun-size Butterfinger
- 1 and ¼ fun-size Baby Ruth
- About 13 pieces of candy corn
- 1 and 1/3 fun-size Heath Bars
- 1 ½ fun-size Hershey Bars
- 1 ½ fun-size Kit Kats
- 10 peanut M&Ms
- 18 plain M&Ms
- 10 peanut butter M&Ms
- 1 and ½ fun-size Mounds bars
- ¾ Reese's Peanut Butter Cup
- 1 and ¼ fun-size Snicker bar
- 1 and 1/8 cup of blueberries
- About 30 dry-roasted pistachios
- 1 scoop of low-fat frozen yogurt
- A little over 2 cups of watermelon
- A little over 9 Kalamata olives
- A little over a 1/3 of a cup of guacamole
- ½ cup slow-churned ice cream
- 6 cups of microwave popcorn, just check the brand
- 14 almonds
- Frozen banana
- 1 and 1/3 eggs
- 2 cups of strawberries

Other Helpful Ideas to Lose Weight and Feel Great

We've all heard them before, only now it's time to take them to heart; because now you have the motivation and the power to make the changes in your life, including your weight goals, that you desire.

Don't mistake thirty for hungry. Drink plenty of water and other low calorie beverages.

Stave off the nighttime munchies by limiting television time. Play a game, read a book or go do something.

Stop with the eating because there is nothing better to do. Find something better to do.

Enjoy the foods you love and stop feeling guilty about it. I love See's candy and I am not going to give it up. I just don't eat it every day. Save up and practice moderation.

Switch sauces for spices.

Don't keep around an abundance of unhealthy food.

Try to eat fresh, rather than packaged, foods.

Sleep enough.

Learn and live portion size.

Stop eating when you are full.

Be careful of empty calories, especially those in alcohol.

Keep your food journal faithfully.

Don't go it alone. Engage family and friends – or me – friend me on Facebook https://www.facebook.com/elizabeth.chapinpinotti or talk to me on my blog http://jumpstartforlife.blogspot.com. Let me help motivate you.

Eat slowly and don't gobble. (I have a tough time with this one)

Push-ups are your friends. (The exercise kind)

Limiting eating out. When you do eat out, watch your portions. Just because they serve it, doesn't mean you have to eat it.

Sauce on the side.

Work thought the discomfort of changing your eating habits. Ask for help if you need it.

Use the wild card days. Indulging isn't bad if it is the exception rather than the rule.

If you are not hungry enough to eat an apple you are not hungry.

A fifteen minute walk after each meal burns 100 calories – or ten peanut M&Ms.

Aim for a realistic size and keep a visual reminder.

Use more vinegar. I have always, always been a vinegar person. I used to drink the bottom of the salad bowl when I was little. Vinegar is amazing. Don't underestimate its use in foods.

Don't subtract foods from your diet – add them. Don't stop eating chocolate, but add beans or peaches to the mix.

A calorie burned is a calorie burned. If you hate working out or dislike the gym – go for a walk, roller blade, garden, walk the golf course, climb a tree – just move.

Take stairs, choose a far parking spot, walk any time you can.

Quit with the starving yourself. Has it worked so far?

Bring your own snacks.

Stand up when you can. You burn about 1.5 times more calories standing than sitting.

Visualize yourself the size you want to be. Think thin.

Eat spicy foods.

Cook your own food, or at least most of it.

Pick your ten favorite low calorie dinners, put them on index cards and use them for your go to meals. We love the burritos. They do well with leftovers and we could eat them everyday.

Use red pepper flakes. They help control appetite and spice up food.

Double recipes and eat leftovers.

Cut back on salt – that means fast food.

If you spend ten minutes per day walking up and down stairs, and don't eat any more or less, you will lose ten pounds.

Skip the salty food aisle in the grocery store or market.

Try to spike all boxed, bagged and packaged foods.

Jot down tips of your own as you discover them:

_____

_____

_____

_____

_____

Real Reasons to Keep a Journal

To stay motivated

To understand your habits.

To keep yourself accountable

To make your goals real.

To see what works.

To see what doesn't work.

To show you are serious about you.

To keep track of what you eat.

To keep track of your progress

To motivate yourself.

Keeping it Going
Staying Started

Food Notes and Other Thoughts for Day _____

_____
_____
_____
_____

Small Steps I've Made: _____

_____
_____
_____
_____
_____

What I ate today:

Breakfast:

_____
_____

Lunch:

_____
_____

Dinner:

_____
_____
_____

Snacks:

_____
_____

Food Notes and Other Thoughts for Day _____

_____
_____
_____
_____

Small Steps I've Made: _____
_____
_____
_____
_____

What I ate today:

Breakfast:
_____
_____

Lunch:
_____
_____

Dinner:
_____
_____
_____

Snacks:
_____
_____

Food Notes and Other Thoughts for Day _____

_____

_____

_____

_____

Small Steps I've Made: _____

_____

_____

_____

_____

What I ate today:

Breakfast:

_____

_____

Lunch:

_____

_____

Dinner:

_____

_____

_____

Snacks:

_____

_____

Food Notes and Other Thoughts for Day _____

_____
_____
_____
_____

Small Steps I've Made: _____
_____
_____
_____
_____
_____

What I ate today:

Breakfast:
_____
_____

Lunch:
_____
_____

Dinner:
_____
_____
_____

Snacks:
_____
_____

Food Notes and Other Thoughts for Day _____

_____

_____

_____

_____

Small Steps I've Made: _____

_____

_____

_____

_____

What I ate today:

Breakfast:

_____

_____

Lunch:

_____

_____

_____

Dinner:

_____

_____

_____

Snacks:

_____

_____

Food Notes and Other Thoughts for Day _____

_____

_____

_____

_____

Small Steps I've Made: _____

_____

_____

_____

_____

What I ate today:

Breakfast:

_____

_____

Lunch:

_____

_____

Dinner:

_____

_____

_____

Snacks:

_____

_____

Food Notes and Other Thoughts for Day _____

_____
_____
_____
_____

Small Steps I've Made: _____

_____
_____
_____
_____

What I ate today:

Breakfast:
_____

Lunch:
_____
_____

Dinner:
_____
_____
_____

Snacks:
_____
_____

Food Notes and Other Thoughts for Day _____

_____

_____

_____

_____

Small Steps I've Made: _____

_____

_____

_____

_____

_____

What I ate today:

Breakfast:

_____

Lunch:

_____

_____

Dinner:

_____

_____

_____

Snacks:

_____

_____

Food Notes and Other Thoughts for Day _____

_____

_____

_____

_____

Small Steps I've Made: _____

_____

_____

_____

_____

What I ate today:

Breakfast:

_____

_____

Lunch:

_____

_____

Dinner:

_____

_____

_____

Snacks:

_____

_____

Food Notes and Other Thoughts for Day _____

_____

_____

_____

_____

Small Steps I've Made: _____

_____

_____

_____

_____

What I ate today:

Breakfast:

_____

Lunch:

_____

_____

Dinner:

_____

_____

Snacks:

_____

_____

Food Notes and Other Thoughts for Day _____

_____

_____

_____

_____

Small Steps I've Made: _____

_____

_____

_____

_____

What I ate today:

Breakfast:

_____

_____

Lunch:

_____

_____

_____

Dinner:

_____

_____

_____

_____

Snacks:

_____

_____

Food Notes and Other Thoughts for Day _____

_____

_____

_____

_____

Small Steps I've Made: _____

_____

_____

_____

_____

What I ate today:

Breakfast:

_____

Lunch:

_____

_____

Dinner:

_____

_____

Snacks:

_____

_____

Food Notes and Other Thoughts for Day _____

_____

_____

_____

_____

Small Steps I've Made: _____

_____

_____

_____

_____

What I ate today:

Breakfast:

_____

_____

Lunch:

_____

_____

Dinner:

_____

_____

_____

Snacks:

_____

_____

Food Notes and Other Thoughts for Day _____

_____

_____

_____

_____

Small Steps I've Made: _____

_____

_____

_____

_____

_____

What I ate today:

Breakfast:

_____

Lunch:

_____

_____

Dinner:

_____

_____

_____

Snacks:

_____

_____

Food Notes and Other Thoughts for Day _____

_____

_____

_____

_____

Small Steps I've Made: _____

_____

_____

_____

_____

What I ate today:

Breakfast:

_____

_____

Lunch:

_____

_____

Dinner:

_____

_____

_____

Snacks:

_____

_____

Food Notes and Other Thoughts for Day _____

_____

_____

_____

_____

Small Steps I've Made: _____

_____

_____

_____

_____

What I ate today:

Breakfast:
_____

Lunch:
_____

_____

Dinner:
_____

_____

_____

Snacks:
_____

_____

Food Notes and Other Thoughts for Day _____

_____

_____

_____

_____

Small Steps I've Made: _____

_____

_____

_____

_____

What I ate today:

Breakfast:

_____

_____

Lunch:

_____

_____

Dinner:

_____

_____

_____

Snacks:

_____

_____

Food Notes and Other Thoughts for Day _____

_____

_____

_____

_____

Small Steps I've Made: _____

_____

_____

_____

_____

What I ate today:

Breakfast:

_____

_____

Lunch:

_____

_____

Dinner:

_____

_____

_____

Snacks:

_____

_____

Food Notes and Other Thoughts for Day _____

_____

_____

_____

_____

Small Steps I've Made: _____

_____

_____

_____

_____

What I ate today:

Breakfast:

_____

Lunch:

_____

_____

Dinner:

_____

_____

_____

Snacks:

_____

_____

Food Notes and Other Thoughts for Day _____

_____
_____
_____
_____

Small Steps I've Made: _____

_____
_____
_____
_____
_____

What I ate today:

Breakfast:

_____
_____

Lunch:

_____
_____

Dinner:

_____
_____
_____

Snacks:

_____
_____

Food Notes and Other Thoughts for Day _____

_____

_____

_____

_____

Small Steps I've Made: _____

_____

_____

_____

_____

What I ate today:

Breakfast:

_____

_____

Lunch:

_____

_____

Dinner:

_____

_____

_____

Snacks:

_____

_____

Food Notes and Other Thoughts for Day _____

_____

_____

_____

_____

Small Steps I've Made: _____

_____

_____

_____

_____

What I ate today:

Breakfast:

_____

Lunch:

_____

_____

Dinner:

_____

_____

Snacks:

_____

_____

Food Notes and Other Thoughts for Day _____

_____

_____

_____

_____

Small Steps I've Made: _____

_____

_____

_____

_____

What I ate today:

Breakfast:

_____

_____

Lunch:

_____

_____

_____

Dinner:

_____

_____

_____

Snacks:

_____

_____

Food Notes and Other Thoughts for Day _____

_____

_____

_____

_____

Small Steps I've Made: _____

_____

_____

_____

_____

What I ate today:

Breakfast:

_____

_____

Lunch:

_____

_____

Dinner:

_____

_____

_____

Snacks:

_____

_____

Food Notes and Other Thoughts for Day _____

_____

_____

_____

_____

Small Steps I've Made: _____

_____

_____

_____

_____

What I ate today:

Breakfast:

_____

_____

Lunch:

_____

_____

Dinner:

_____

_____

_____

Snacks:

_____

_____

Food Notes and Other Thoughts for Day _____

_____

_____

_____

_____

Small Steps I've Made: _____

_____

_____

_____

_____

_____

What I ate today:

Breakfast:

_____

Lunch:

_____

_____

Dinner:

_____

_____

_____

Snacks:

_____

_____

Food Notes and Other Thoughts for Day _____

_____

_____

_____

_____

Small Steps I've Made: _____

_____

_____

_____

_____

What I ate today:

Breakfast:

_____

_____

Lunch:

_____

_____

_____

Dinner:

_____

_____

_____

Snacks:

_____

_____

Food Notes and Other Thoughts for Day _____

_____

_____

_____

_____

Small Steps I've Made: _____

_____

_____

_____

_____

_____

What I ate today:

Breakfast:

_____

Lunch:

_____

_____

Dinner:

_____

_____

_____

Snacks:

_____

_____

Food Notes and Other Thoughts for Day _____

_____

_____

_____

_____

Small Steps I've Made: _____

_____

_____

_____

_____

What I ate today:

Breakfast:

_____

_____

Lunch:

_____

_____

Dinner:

_____

_____

_____

Snacks:

_____

_____

Food Notes and Other Thoughts for Day _____

_____

_____

_____

_____

Small Steps I've Made: _____

_____

_____

_____

_____

What I ate today:

Breakfast:

_____

_____

Lunch:

_____

_____

Dinner:

_____

_____

_____

Snacks:

_____

_____

Food Notes and Other Thoughts for Day _____

_____

_____

_____

_____

Small Steps I've Made: _____

_____

_____

_____

_____

_____

What I ate today:

Breakfast:

_____

_____

Lunch:

_____

_____

Dinner:

_____

_____

_____

Snacks:

_____

_____

Food Notes and Other Thoughts for Day _____

_____

_____

_____

_____

Small Steps I've Made: _____

_____

_____

_____

_____

What I ate today:

Breakfast:

_____

Lunch:

_____

_____

Dinner:

_____

_____

Snacks:

_____

_____

Food Notes and Other Thoughts for Day _____

_____

_____

_____

_____

Small Steps I've Made: _____

_____

_____

_____

_____

What I ate today:

Breakfast:

_____

_____

Lunch:

_____

_____

Dinner:

_____

_____

_____

Snacks:

_____

_____

Food Notes and Other Thoughts for Day _____

_____

_____

_____

_____

Small Steps I've Made: _____

_____

_____

_____

_____

What I ate today:

Breakfast:

_____

Lunch:

_____

_____

Dinner:

_____

_____

Snacks:

_____

_____

Food Notes and Other Thoughts for Day _____

_____

_____

_____

_____

Small Steps I've Made: _____

_____

_____

_____

_____

What I ate today:

Breakfast:

_____

_____

Lunch:

_____

_____

Dinner:

_____

_____

_____

Snacks:

_____

_____

Food Notes and Other Thoughts for Day _____

_____

_____

_____

_____

Small Steps I've Made: _____

_____

_____

_____

_____

What I ate today:

Breakfast:

_____

Lunch:

_____

_____

Dinner:

_____

_____

_____

Snacks:

_____

_____

Food Notes and Other Thoughts for Day _____

_____
_____
_____
_____

Small Steps I've Made: _____

_____
_____
_____
_____
_____

What I ate today:

Breakfast:

_____
_____

Lunch:

_____
_____
_____

Dinner:

_____
_____
_____

Snacks:

_____
_____

Food Notes and Other Thoughts for Day _____

_____

_____

_____

_____

Small Steps I've Made: _____

_____

_____

_____

_____

What I ate today:

Breakfast:

_____

Lunch:

_____

_____

Dinner:

_____

_____

_____

Snacks:

_____

_____

Food Notes and Other Thoughts for Day _____

_____

_____

_____

_____

Small Steps I've Made: _____

_____

_____

_____

_____

What I ate today:

Breakfast:

_____

_____

Lunch:

_____

_____

Dinner:

_____

_____

_____

Snacks:

_____

_____

Food Notes and Other Thoughts for Day _____

_____

_____

_____

_____

Small Steps I've Made: _____

_____

_____

_____

_____

What I ate today:

Breakfast:

_____

_____

Lunch:

_____

_____

Dinner:

_____

_____

_____

Snacks:

_____

_____

Food Notes and Other Thoughts for Day _____

_____

_____

_____

_____

Small Steps I've Made: _____

_____

_____

_____

_____

What I ate today:

Breakfast:

_____

_____

Lunch:

_____

_____

Dinner:

_____

_____

_____

_____

Snacks:

_____

_____

Food Notes and Other Thoughts for Day _____

_____

_____

_____

_____

Small Steps I've Made: _____

_____

_____

_____

_____

What I ate today:

Breakfast:

_____

Lunch:

_____

_____

Dinner:

_____

_____

_____

Snacks:

_____

_____

Food Notes and Other Thoughts for Day _____

_____

_____

_____

_____

Small Steps I've Made: _____

_____

_____

_____

_____

What I ate today:

Breakfast:

_____

Lunch:

_____

_____

Dinner:

_____

_____

_____

Snacks:

_____

_____

Food Notes and Other Thoughts for Day _____

_____

_____

_____

_____

Small Steps I've Made: _____

_____

_____

_____

_____

What I ate today:

Breakfast:

_____

_____

Lunch:

_____

_____

Dinner:

_____

_____

_____

Snacks:

_____

_____

Food Notes and Other Thoughts for Day _____

_____

_____

_____

_____

Small Steps I've Made: _____

_____

_____

_____

_____

What I ate today:

Breakfast:

_____

Lunch:

_____

_____

Dinner:

_____

_____

_____

Snacks:

_____

_____

Food Notes and Other Thoughts for Day _____

_____

_____

_____

_____

Small Steps I've Made: _____

_____

_____

_____

_____

What I ate today:

Breakfast:

_____

Lunch:

_____

_____

Dinner:

_____

_____

Snacks:

_____

_____

Food Notes and Other Thoughts for Day _____

_____

_____

_____

_____

Small Steps I've Made: _____

_____

_____

_____

_____

What I ate today:

Breakfast:

_____

Lunch:

_____

_____

Dinner:

_____

_____

_____

Snacks:

_____

_____

Food Notes and Other Thoughts for Day _____

_____

_____

_____

_____

Small Steps I've Made: _____

_____

_____

_____

_____

What I ate today:

Breakfast:

_____

_____

Lunch:

_____

_____

_____

Dinner:

_____

_____

_____

Snacks:

_____

_____

Food Notes and Other Thoughts for Day _____

_____

_____

_____

_____

Small Steps I've Made: _____

_____

_____

_____

_____

What I ate today:

Breakfast:

_____

Lunch:

_____

_____

Dinner:

_____

_____

Snacks:

_____

_____